T0172435

WILD ONION NURSE

WILD ONION NURSE

A collection of 25 years of the poetry of nursing in a college of medicine literary journal

JUDY SCHAEFER

Radcliffe Publishing
Oxford • New York

Radcliffe Publishing Ltd
18 Marcham Road
Abingdon
Oxon OX14 1AA
United Kingdom

www.radcliffe-oxford.com
Electronic catalogue and worldwide online ordering facility.

British Library Cataloguing in Publication Data

A catalogue record for this book is available from the British Library.

ISBN-13: 978 184619 417 7

Typeset by Pindar NZ, Auckland, New Zealand
Printed and bound by Cadmus Communications, USA

For my grandsons,
W. Conor Lenhardt and Noah P. Lenhardt.

J.S.

Contents

8 CONTENTS

About the Author

Judy Schaefer, RNC, MA is editor of the first autobiographical/biographical volume about nurse–poets, *The Poetry of Nursing* (Kent State University Press, 2006), and a pioneering co-editor, with Cortney Davis, of the first international anthology of creative writing by nurses, *Between the Heartbeats* (University of Iowa Press, 1995), followed by *Intensive Care* (University of Iowa Press, 2003), the second anthology by Davis and Schaefer. She is the author of a collection of poetry, *Harvesting the Dew* (Vista, 1997). Judy has lectured for the Pennsylvania State University and is a member of The Kienle Center, Penn State University, College of Medicine, Hershey, PA.

Judy is east coast poetry editor for *PULSE: voices from the heart of medicine,* an electronic online literary journal, and the poetry editor of *24/7/365 International Journal of Healthcare and Humanities,* a scholarly journal that stimulates creativity, scholarship, and compassion, which is produced at Penn State College of Medicine Department of Humanities. Judy can be reached by visiting her website at www.judyschaefer.biz or contacting her by email at jschaefer@mindspring.com.

Permissions and Acknowledgments

"Of Repression and Archeology", "Hey, Lady That Hurts Like Hell", "Intensive Care Waiting Room", "She Was Raped", "Bag Lady", "Windfall Apples", "Sundance", "Primary Care", and "On Being Passed By a Class of Medical Students While Seated" were published in *Harvesting the Dew* (Vista, 1997).

"Intensive Care Waiting Room" was published in *The Arduous Touch*, edited by A. Haddad and K. Brown (Purdue University Press, 1999).

"Seeing My Grandson for the First Time" and "A Welcome to a Second Grandson" were published as one poem, "A Pediatric Nurse Over Time", in *Intensive Care*, edited by C. Davis and J. Schaefer (University of Iowa Press, 2003).

"Feather and Claw", "Long Hospital Stay", "Medicine from the Wood", and "Who Owns the Libretto?" were published in *Between the Heartbeats*, edited by C. Davis and J. Schaefer (University of Iowa Press, 1995).

"Who Owns the Libretto?" was published in *Clinician Reviews*, Vol. 7, No. 9, in September 1997.

All of the poems in this collection were first published by *Wild Onions*, which has returned copyright to the author.

Special acknowledgement and gratitude are expressed to Joanne

Trautmann Banks, Anne Hunsaker-Hawkins, and Doctors Jane and Lawrence Kienle, whose efforts have made *Wild Onions* and my poetic voice possible. Thank you!

Introduction

"Write two poems and call me in the morning" – unlikely advice, isn't it? How about the 65-year-old woman, who has been living alone and independently until now, waiting on a gurney in the emergency room with a fractured hip: "Read three poems by Wallace Stevens and one short story by Raymond Carver." Not quite! Please call in the orthopedic surgeon!

While, indeed, poetry "read" and poetry "written" have a healing component, poetry is a literary art form, not a medical or nursing prescription. However, poetry and creative writing by nurses can be especially revealing in a healthcare system that is burdened by cost and regulation. My state test and my state license are not enough to ensure that I will practice at my highest level. Numerous local and federal agencies monitor, audit and accredit the work of myself and others in the healthcare system. Not bad, but not necessarily good – many of the regulations are boggy and burdensome.

Creative writing has provided a place for me to take my frustration and my joy. My writing is an art and an outlet, as writing is for other nurses. *Visions of War, Dreams of Peace*, a collection of creative writing by women in the Vietnam War edited by two nurses, Lynda Van Devanter and Joan A. Furey (New York: Warner Books, 1991), was the beginning of *Zeitgeistic* writing by nurses. Cortney Davis and I followed with our international anthology of nurse-only writing in

Between the Heartbeats (Iowa City: University of Iowa Press, 1995).
Then came Amy Marie Haddad and Kate H. Brown, *The Arduous Touch, Women's Voices in Health Care*, including nurses (West Lafayette, Indiana: Purdue University Press, 1999). Meanwhile, numerous nurses were writing up a storm with novels, poetry and essays, sometimes identifying themselves as nurses and sometimes not. With the Kent State University Press, I have been privileged to publish a biographical/autobiographical book about 14 nurses who are prolific poets, *The Poetry of Nursing* (Kent, Ohio: Kent State University Press, 2006).

Wild Onions, although not consistently published each year, was a welcome oasis for my poetry in 1984. While it was a literary journal for and by the Pennsylvania State University College of Medicine students mentored by Joanne Trautmann Banks, I stumbled upon it and was welcomed in. At the time, I knew no other nurses who were writing as seriously as I was attempting to write. The *Wild Onions* title is explained as follows in the journal:

> The wild onion is a common garden variety weed, a hardy plant that grows almost anywhere and tends to spring up in unexpected places throughout the woods and fields and roadsides in this part of the country. It blossoms into an unusual purple flower and its underground bulk, if tasted, yields a pungent, spicy flavor. The wild onion is a symbol of the commonplace yet surprising beauty that is living and growing around us all the time, the spice that though uncultivated, unexpectedly thrives and – if we only take time to notice – enhances life.

I am grateful to *Wild Onions*, and to The Doctors Kienle Center for Humanistic Medicine at Pennsylvania State University College of Medicine, for the continued support of this literary vehicle for myself and for increasingly more nurses. My 24/7/365 nurse–poet voice found a home here, and has thrived for 25 years and more.

My first poem was published in *Wild Onions* in 1984. Amongst the hallways and byways of the Medical Center I had picked up a copy of *Wild Onions*, and I asked around until I found these medical students and residents who were publishing the literary journal. As an admitted print-addictive I have read everything that I could find from the time I was a child. The whole concept of the mystery of words as a code to be explored and excavated was a deep and broad archeological field. The process of words and language is still an awesome mystery to me.

The poem from 1984 reminds me of my transformation from a country girl with pigtails, born on a farm in Southeast Missouri, to a young striving professional on the streets of St. Louis. I recall, even now, the pleasure of being filled with energy, breakfast, and words – in this case *The New York Times*. My future was bubbling and frothing inside my mind and muscles ready to be – the future could be – golden. My energy and my dreams were wonderful secrets that I wanted to release. I desired transformation. What would I think of this poem 25 years later?

As a youngster on a farm, I loved animals and they were natural companions. Beyond companionship, the cats and dogs had their jobs to do. The cats kept the mice and rats away, and the dogs barked and protected when danger, or at least something unusual, came to our gates and doors. One special black and white dog, whose name was Buster, was the hunting partner of my father (Coy Welker). Recollection of Buster's death is an image of the reality of country life. Buster was old and ill, and death was imminent. Five miles off the paved highway on a wooded farm in the foothills of the Ozarks, there was no vet to euthanize him. My father picked up his shot gun and Buster's tail began to wag in anticipation of a day of hunting; they walked into the woods and Dad placed a bullet, swiftly, accurately, and just once into Buster's head.

My brother and I waited on the back porch. We heard the shot. Years later as a nurse, I could be expected to know a level of comfort in the realities of life and death. Not so. I was not any better prepared than any of my classmates.

It was over. My Dad, while stoic on this occasion, was a gentleman with a soft voice, a sensitive nature, an easy smile, and a big wide country laugh. He loved and knew intimately each and every animal on the farm. He knew and respected their personalities, and especially loved his horses. He knew life and he knew death as intimate partners. Do not get me wrong, but get me right on this – he was a kind man, but a strong and self-sufficient man, as many farmers were and are today. It was over. He came in for supper and sat down with my mother (Lettie Loberg Welker). Life went on. My mother was a creative and supportive helpmate. Her beautiful singing voice filled the house and the large one-acre kitchen garden. I am not sure she sang from happiness, but I always sensed that she sang to remind herself that she had a voice – that her vocal cords were alive. Often when I write, I seek her voice – to give her honor and to hear her once again. And to love her.

Farmers, by the nature of their work, always seem to know how to do what must be done. I love the self-sufficient nature and earth-knowledge skill of farmers. Not surprisingly, when I write of self-sufficiency, I write of my father.

I was fortunate to have the run of a farm, its fields, meadows, and woods, until the age of eight years. I was further fortunate to have a brother, five years older, who watched and protected my every step. We lived on a cultural cusp, which later I would recognize as an enrichment of every thought and action that I would take into the future. I feel fortunate to be old enough to have had these experiences, but young enough to make use of modernity and this computer on which I write these words.

The experience of electricity and what could happen with the flip of a switch arrived when I was five years old. Until then we used wood for cooking and heating, and we used coal oil lamps at night for reading (kerosene as recovered from coal, hence the name "coal oil"). I recall the anticipation and excitement of the "high lines" coming through the woods. A path was carved out from tall timber, and the forest was separated like the proverbial sea for the magical lines on high poles. My brother, our cousins, and I were enchanted, perhaps in the same way that a child might be enchanted the first time they see Disney World. Our imaginative experience was not unlike the experiences of Charlotte, Emily, Anne, and Branwell Brontë in Haworth, Yorkshire, or the fictional experience of Tom Sawyer in Hannibal, Missouri. The absence of experience was, in itself, the canvas on which a vast imaginative experience could be played out as only children can play.

The magical lines would bring lights and would be followed by television a few years later. And even later, microwave ovens. My father, at the age of 90, stood in front of his microwave and said one day, "I know it works but I don't know how it works. It is a mystery to me." In that quick moment an image was split of forebearers over fire and of future generations using microwaves and new technologies beyond the wildest dreams of my father. I felt a split, a rip, through my consciousness, moving from fire, wheels, and food from the earth. The new vortex was a transformation into a new and as yet unimagined world. Our grandsons will imagine it and produce it someday.

Until the debut of electricity through the tall ancient trees, we had huddled at night around the radio and the coal oil lamps. We told stories and talked about the adventures of our day. We took the frail threads of daily life and wove them into a rich and vibrant carpet of the imagination. We believed in God and in each other and reaffirmed this each night. Our heritage was German and Irish, and to this very day, this storytelling and talk is what I love about Ireland. There is no doubt that I feel right at home when in Ireland.

Yet I must say that, too, is the "old" Ireland. Ireland, like America, long ago moved into the high-tech wilderness of the twenty-first century. While tourists are drawn to Ireland because of the kindest of the people and the pubs and the quaintness of the cottages and the small white lambs in the green fields, Ireland is and has been on the cutting edge of technology.

If I did not live here – I do love America and its rugged history – I would choose Ireland. The love of language and the accuracy in the use of language in Ireland draws me there, in addition to the near supernatural feeling of being in the right place when I am there, the place where I was meant to be. My family history is in fact filled with family stories and family records of an Irish relative by the name of Timothy Reagan (born in 1750), who fought in the Revolutionary

War and was wounded at Brandywine on 11 September 1777, as was Lafayette. Apparently, after a long recovery, he returned to battle and was wounded again in the war. There are members of our family who like to think that we are related to President Reagan, but I have not found any documentation to support this.

Timothy Reagan's grandfather, another Timothy Reagan (born in 1678), apparently came to Anne Arundel County, Maryland, from Ireland in the late 1600s and married Mary O'Leary at St. Margaret's Parish in Anne Arundel County in 1703. Mary O'Leary's history is unknown to me or, should I say, is as yet undiscovered. Please note that Timothy was apparently a very popular name within the family.

Once on this side of the Atlantic, most records place these early Reagans in Western Anne Arundel County near Elkridge and near Charles Carroll's plantation, Doughoragen Manor, not far from Baltimore. Yes, Dough*oragen*. Charles Carroll (born in 1660) came to America from England and Ireland in 1688. It is likely that the Reagans were tenants or servants of Charles Carroll and might have come to America with his assistance. His grandson, Charles Carroll (born in 1737) signed the Declaration of Independence and was the last signer of the Declaration to die, in 1832 at the age of 95 years. This longevity is pretty unusual. Relatives of Charles Carroll still live in Doughoragen Manor, one of the oldest family homes in Maryland.

I have not discovered the original immigrant Timothy's Irish home or his or his family's reason for leaving, or the date of their leaving. One can guess at land loss and Cromwell. Name places surface like Kilmichael Parish not so far from Michael Skellig. The reader can quickly see how nebulous the research becomes once the documentation and the oral history start to fade. Logic suggests that the point of departure was from Cobh Harbor in County Cork in Southern Ireland. These trips to America were long and arduous, taking from one and a half to two months. I cannot imagine the fear and the determination of those who chose to board those ships and leave everything behind. Many, of course, did not survive the long sea voyage.

Some 100 years later, Irish immigrants would board ships at

Cobh Harbor to escape the famine in Ireland by going to America, Australia, England, and Europe and other destinations. The fear of these famine travellers, too, is beyond my imagination. There is no comparison to the six-hour trip on Aer Lingus Airlines that one can make today.

When I think of these Irish immigrants in colonial times or famine times, I cannot help but think of them as "travaillers." What travails! What toil! What pain!

Although the Internet has made genealogy research easier, limitations persist because of lack of my own time and lack of resources and documentation. There is so much I don't know – so much still to be discovered.

What I do know is that Timothy Reagan's grandson, Richard Rainwater Reagan (born in 1828 in Tennessee), migrated to Missouri in 1834 with his parents and married Rutha Caroline Mills (born in 1832) in 1850. Their daughter Rutha Caroline Reagan (born in 1865) would become my great grandmother. She married James Welker (born in 1859) in 1883, and my grandfather, Pola Welker, was born in 1884.

(Richard Rainwater Reagan died on 16 January 1897; 16 January 1912 would be my father's birth date, and 16 January 1997 would be the birth date of one of our grandsons. What is it with these numbers?)

When my grandfather, Pola, a blonde blue-eyed toddler, was about 5 years old, his mother was pregnant again, but was to die in childbirth, and the newborn was to die soon afterwards. This left Pola alone with his father. The story has existed for years within the family that his mother's older brother, his Uncle George Reagan, offered to take his nephew and raise him. Apparently and naturally there was some resistance, but not much, on the part of Pola's father. In all fairness, James Welker's story was never fully told, or at least I never heard it. It was my grandfather's story as told by my father and others that held my attention. I would ask to hear the story over and over again. That is what we did with stories – we repeated them in much the same way that children today watch their favorite videos over and over again.

My father always told their story from the perspective of my grandfather choosing between uncle and father. The story goes that they were at a public event, an auction, and Uncle George, who was sitting on his black horse, looked down and asked his tiny nephew if he wanted to come and live with him. My grandfather, looking up, said "Yes", and was at once pulled up onto the horse behind his Uncle George. And off they went. End of story.

In today's context, this is a fascinating version of the story of a child allowed to choose, and of a child's wise decision. The basis for the toddler's wisdom, in my Dad's view, lay in the peripheral stories of James Welker's happy-go-lucky nature and George Reagan's stable nature. The story's congruence for me was my grandfather Pola's personality. He was resilient and wise in my view. He sang or whistled while he went off to the barn; he smiled and hummed while he stroked the neck of one of his horses. He stood tall with a straight and proud backbone. Neighbors and relatives would ask for and respect his opinion. While apparently no relation of former President Reagan, imagine my grandfather as well as my father in the same physical framework – tall, handsome, horse-loving storytellers with an even temperament and easy laugh. And my father and grandfather were slow to anger, but once they were angered that anger was white hot.

(Resources for my family history have been the primary resources of stories from my father and other family members as well as conventional wisdom. Several books have been helpful. There are five self-published books, namely *Reagan History, from the Smokies to the Ozarks, 1834–1993*, by Willa Reagan Combs and Rudy Reagan (1993), *The Book of Ragan/Reagan*, by Donald B. Reagan (1993), and *Smoky Mountain Clans, Volumes 1, 2 and 3*, by Donald B. Reagan (1974, 1978, and 1983). A book that provided powerful insight and background information is *Princes of Ireland, Planters of Maryland: A Carroll Saga, 1500–1782*, written by Ronald Hoffman in collaboration with Sally D. Mason, and published by the University of North Carolina Press in 2000.)

1 9 8 4

OPENINGS/COMING ATTRACTIONS

I walked this morning
 on the streets
before the shops were open
Early
Yet I'd already had
 Breakfast and the New York Times
I looked at myself in mirrors
windows dark from inside
My image wavered
 Lines hung in time
Movements of shopkeepers
 Stocking
 Stacking
Quietly   Acts unseen
 Discreetly

 As if they had
 a secret to hide
to be unlocked at nine

HE'S GLAD TO HAVE ME BACK

His engine hums at my shoes
His neck strokes my ankles
    as I shed my stockings
I hobble, nearly topple
I try not to catch his tail
Glad to be home but unbalanced underfoot
    by his motorized welcome
He follows me to the shower
on stealthy gray flannel pads
and catches stray drops of water
He doesn't ease into his warm content
    circle of down
until my packing's undone
My feet up, unstocked, unshoed
My hair loosened and brushed out
Now every feline piece of fur can be put
    into place

OF REPRESSION AND ARCHEOLOGY

I watch myself
bury memories in my brain
like a dog
buries bones in the ground
Furious splatter
of earth and gray matter
Eyes on guard
Secretly
What will strike the discord
Hungry trigger
of some primitive instinct
To dig

Pain observed and pain inflicted for good are part of good nursing. Movements and fads in nursing and medicine come and go. One such "movement" was the use of hypnosis and relaxation techniques. We all tried it, and still do in some cases, I suppose. "Hey, Lady That Hurts Like Hell" is an attempt to describe the reality. The techniques did not always work.

Life and death are always present in the wards. Life is that spunky, sometimes sexy, energetic presence, and death, as I saw it in "Intensive Care Waiting Room," is that gray vapor which snakes about those working and those waiting in the Intensive Care Unit.

In "I Once Heard That the Bones of Birds Are Hollow" I anticipated what I feel now. It makes me feel curious and goosebumpy to look back at the accuracy of the poem. If I do say so myself, it holds up pretty well. And I do tremble at the recall of those red hot days of lust and energy. To make love is just not accurate – to make lust is a more accurate way to describe the parties, the alcohol, the laughter, the loud music, and the exchanges that occurred at the end of the day – at the end of the shift and sometimes in the supply closet. There is nothing quite like lusty sex to remind you that, in the midst of death, you are pulsatingly alive.

The point is that lust is a life force. In the midst of death, lust is the door left open, a way out of the fear. Nothing like a good snug – a good frontal snug – with the sound of a vent breathing and a pump clicking in the background. Scrubs and nursing uniforms are made of thin material. Ah, there it was, the ease and safety of zipless fucks.

The term "zipless fuck" was coined in the era before AIDS by Erica Jong in her novel *Fear of Flying* (published in 1973). Sex on the wards was solid functional lust at its best, with promises of some kind of love at the end of the week. The promise was rarely kept, and the promise was rarely believed in any case. The baseness of lust was about getting through the moment and making it through the horrors and stench of a night on the wards.

Well, enough about sex. This collection is dedicated to my grandsons after all.

And, of course, lust isn't love. Love is on a higher plane and enjoys trust, faithfulness, passion, vision, comradeship, and, of course – yes, of course – lots of passion with visions of a future together. But dare I try to define love?

There is nothing quite like a husband, children, grandchildren, and friends and a long life filled with meaning to remind you that you will not die in your own narrow arms. I am grateful for all the support over all the years from my husband, Dan. He has helped me to keep "a room of my own", and he keeps a garden and cooks. He supports my poetry, even when he doesn't understand exactly what I am trying to say.

And we travel well together. Dan tends to be the talker and I tend to be the texter. He solves problems by talking about them, and I solve problems by reading or writing about them. I read and follow the signs, and he talks and asks for directions. He is, in fact, not at all afraid to ask for directions because it gives him an opportunity to have a little chat – or as it so often works out in Ireland – a nice afternoon-long chat.

1987

"HEY, LADY THAT HURTS LIKE HELL"

Let's be a good patient
while we slip this piece of silver steel
    into our vein
Icy glide through red serpent canal
Let's not say pain, let's say hurt
Pain's not pain if given another name
Or so it was said in our relaxation classes
We call it discomfort, pressure, sting
Just think of blue skies and warm sandy beaches
or if you prefer, warm yellow haystacks
Just think sweetly and relax
We know everything, we've read the books
We've had the course

Oops!
Silver steel pop
Red burst canal
Over the side
Off course
White knuckle shore

Now we know we didn't do this quite right
and we'll go home with a pink hematoma
And we'll turn purple overnight
And we'll turn yellow green
by the end of the week
Let's be a good patient

INTENSIVE CARE WAITING ROOM

The gray vapor of death
reaches into the enclave
like infinite snakes of fog
Mocking teasing striking
Moving always moving
Turning flipping turning
Striking
Slithering around ankles
Passing touching soft tissue of faces
A caress
Offering a terminal final promise
Loving coaxing fluttering
in a stagnant cave
Stones blocking exit or entry
Striking
And on another floor in another room
a baby cries with a first surprise
first gasp of father's air
And on another floor in another room
a young man flirts
and walks on a virgin wooden leg
He winks and calls the leg Margaret
And on another floor in another room
a sallow nurse
pulls tight the sterile
sheets on a freshly made bed
like ice across a white pond
And a maid down a tunnel
moves thin shoulders hips hands
according to aseptic technique
Striking
They huddle and wait
and they wait
according to the gray rules of death

I ONCE HEARD THAT THE BONES OF BIRDS ARE HOLLOW

I once heard that the bones of birds are hollow
I once thought spring the season
    with all merit
    Surging forth
    Growing up
    Budding, pink blooming and leafed green
But perhaps it is autumn
    The cooling off
    Settling in
                    Banking up
    Storing, savoring walnuts and red wine
Yet there will be the frosted panes of winter
    The looking back
    Cradling my own
    white marrow bones
    Warming at the red fire
of lazy crackling dreams of summers gone
    And I, I tremble
    at recall
    of those red hot days
    And fear dying in my own narrow arms

As a woman and as a nurse – I had no control over the first and I chose the latter. In the 1960s and into the 1980s gender inequities continued. I fought these battles as much as I could while trying to maintain my employment and my dignity. I wanted to solve this situation for myself as well as for my daughter. This was easier said than done. When I saw promotion and the bigger pay check go to the guy because he had a wife and family, it felt like rape. When I went home to my daughter, who had let herself in an hour earlier with a latchkey, it felt like rape.

For a while, before Dan came into our life, I was a single mother because of divorce, and divorce was my choice. So I don't regret my choice because I know for what reason I made the decision. Yet I unwittingly put myself and my child in a vulnerable position. Unfortunately, I suspect not too much has changed. I am older now and have been remarried for 25 plus years. Yet my heart still breaks at our vulnerability in those days.

My past and my experience on the farm did not help. Male and female were so well defined there in the animal population and in my parents and my uncles and aunts. My father and mother were a team, doing clearly differentiated tasks. Dan and I once went on a horse pack trip into the wilderness of Montana, and I learned then of the teamwork required and the negotiation necessary between man and woman. There were instances when I, not being a horsewoman, just really needed his physical strength to help move me from the top of a boulder to the top of a tall horse, or to hammer in the stakes of the tent.

At any rate, back in the early days I did not see any of the challenges of equality and the women's movement coming. I was just happy to have a pay check, and my parents seemed proud of me, and my daughter was healthy and pretty. What more was there?

And then, like a sledge hammer, it hit me. Once my eyes and ears were opened to all that was going on around me, I became slowly but surely enraged. I have always valued privacy, and never thought another person's salary or job description were any of my business. Then I heard Gloria Steinem. I recall seeing her on television as I was passing through the room. She was talking about the value of homemaking and the value of working in the world of commerce. Why were they different? Were they different? Were some jobs thought to be the primary work of women? I started thinking, then seeing and hearing, as if for the first time.

It became cathartic to write about my "sisters." I felt that we had become so sane and our vision was so clear that we were insane with our insight, somewhat like witches of the past. Once there is the "knowing" there is no return to ordinary thinking. As in the poem, "Healing the Heart", the wound persists.

1988

TOO SANE SISTERS

I screech through the black sky
    with the smoky witches of Salem
I covet the slice of moon
    tempered and pounded
    and thin
It cuts clouds with sharp edges
    tarnished silver blade
    crescent
Cutting tool I cannot
    hold, but I reach for it
    and stretch
And bleed with the witches
    profiled in the light at Stonehenge

SHE WAS RAPED

Raped!
Torn glued cut pasted
Paper doll cut from wax paper
Limp pink white stained paper legs
And raped again!
Judge and trial
victim, thighs pried apart in a witness box
Paper doll cut torn glued and pasted
Did you scream?
Did you kick?
Did you fight back?
Did you know him?
Did you flirt?
How many lovers have you had?

She wears colored scarves on her head
Then moves out of town
        and changes her name
Droops and rounds her shoulders to protect her breasts
        and walks with a limp when she wears high heels
He returns to his daughters and wife
complaining about the cold meat
        and throws the plate across the room
And tells how he was prick teased
in the bar that night
How he was drunk
How she asked for it
How it should be a lesson
He tells her every night

But the camera caught his face
Caught him between a practice thought
        split second black and white
Newspaper open on the stoop

She sometimes cries and doesn't know why

HEALING THE HEART

She looks lazy and relaxed
Rather like an invalid
with a leg wound, the white gauze
covered by a green plaid wool rug
who sits on the sun deck for hours at a time

There she sits on a wooden deck
Clings to it like she might hold to a skeleton
watching for unexpected life from dry wood
Looking for fire from splinters
Trying to heal, exposed to the morning sun
She chides herself
for not getting up
There are letters to write
Calls to make and laundry settled in the wicker basket
She has people and places
and tasks to attend
And another cup of tea, she could have
But there she sits
with a green plaid wool rug
pulled up over her wounded heart

THE FIELDS OF FEBRUARY

The fields of February
    are like the creviced stubbled face of an old man
Patches of snow like skin cancer hang on the hills
    that Pennsylvanians call mountains
Roadways are clogged like arteries
    with plaques of cinders
    and salty sludge
If dropped here from another planet place and time
One would not recognize
    this as the dawn of spring

As I read these poems, as a collection, I am slightly uncomfortable with their revealing autobiographical nature. I must go and talk to Dan and see how comfortable he is with what I write.

He chuckles as I start to ask my question. I first seek sympathy and seriousness. I complain of knee pain that I think originates from the strange position from which I read in a couple of my favorite plump leather chairs. In each and every room of our house I have a chair that is comfortable enough for reading. Anyway, my habit is to hang both knees over the arm of the chair and read. While engrossed in the book, my arthritic knee goes into near contracture. My left knee hurts. I gather his sympathy to me like a bouquet of red roses that he offers slowly and liberally one by one.

But I don't know if he has really paid attention to the question I am asking. He kisses me quickly. He, the crusty old athlete, then laughs that I have a "reading" injury. As he goes out of the door to join his foursome, he is still laughing, "Write. Write. You know you have my permission." He is still laughing, "A reading injury!"

"A reading injury. Wait until they hear this one – a reading injury!"

While I write from my imagination and see poetry as a work of art, I understand more than ever that creative art is almost always autobiographical, even when the artist is wildly imaginative. These poems certainly mirror the pain, joy and fatigue of nursing and of living. The poems here are in the order in which they appeared in *Wild Onions*. It was not my intent to write poems for a collection. I was just thrilled beyond my imagination to get a poem published in 1984. There is no order relative to when they were written and when they were published, and as all writers fully understand there is no synchronization anyway with regard to when a poem is written and when it gets published, if it ever does.

I am not sure where I was going with "Bag Lady", but there is a weariness in the poem and a desire perhaps to have nothing but a warm coat and a book of poems. You know, to go forth in the world without responsibility but with clarity, and just watch the world go by. There were those moments when homelessness and poverty seemed unrealistically romantic. The operative word is "unrealistic."

In 1990, the poem "Windfall Apples" surfaces to record the emotions associated with caring for patients with hemophilia. In 1981, nine years prior to the publication of this poem, the first patient with a genetic bleeding disorder in the USA contracted AIDS (acquired immune deficiency syndrome). My first hands-on experience was in 1981, and most of my nursing career has been in advocacy with this community. I, along with my patients and colleagues, was shocked and scared.

Hemophilia is a genetic coagulation disorder that most often looks like a chronic orthopedic problem because it causes bleeding into joint spaces. People with hemophilia can bleed spontaneously as well as in response to trauma. Most hemophilia cases that are treated usually present in one of two varieties, hemophilia A and hemophilia B, although there are rarer types. Hemophilia A is caused by a deficiency or absence of the coagulation protein Factor VIII, and hemophilia B is caused by a deficiency or absence of Factor IX. Hemophilia is a recessive sex-linked genetic disorder. The gene for hemophilia A and B is carried on the X chromosome. Thus conventional wisdom at the time suggested that there were then approximately 20,000 males with hemophilia in the USA, and probably half of them were infected.

We soon learned that the AIDS virus, HIV, was present in the concentrate that people with hemophilia infused on a regular basis to treat life and limb-threatening hemorrhages. Investigators at the Centers for Disease Control (CDC) in Atlanta, Georgia, as well as everyone else, were concluding early on that AIDS was transmitted like hepatitis in the blood supply. This supply was the lifeline for people with hemophilia. The blood supply came from paid and volunteer donors. Now in 2009 the biotechnology is much improved, with safe non-human-derived proteins available for infusion for these individuals.

It was soon learned that AIDS in general was transmitted through bodily fluids such as blood and semen. Blood transfusions and sex were now more than suspect.

I feared AIDS. I continued my nursing practice, and learned to wear gloves as I drew blood and when I infused the factor concentrate into the patient's arm. I embraced universal precautions. Memories of past splashes of blood and needlestick injuries passed through my mind like an aurora borealis in a night-time sky.

One of the doctors (and maybe others, for all I know) would be appalled when I single-handedly decided to distribute condoms in our clinic. I would learn more than I wanted – that doctors and nurses are just human with ordinary fears. Decades had passed since doctors and nurses had been faced with a disease that would test their dedication and willingness to take on some personal risk in order to care for others. Discussions, both formal and informal, would ensue about the amount of risk one should be expected to take, and about the reason why one became a nurse or a doctor in the first place. It was ironic, but those on the periphery, those who did not have their hands and bodies in the trenches of blood and human flesh, but who spoke and wrote from a polished desk, had the most articulate opinions and knew just exactly how we should conduct ourselves.

I gravitated towards the surgeons and particularly towards the orthopedic surgeons on our team in these discussions. Short with words, like good mechanics, the orthopedic surgeons just kept doing what they usually did and kept our patients motoring along. I suppose I shall always have a fondness for the strong bearded image of Surgeon General C. Everett Koop. In October 1986, Koop recommended condoms to reduce the spread of AIDS. I took Koop's words as a mandate.

My small courage surprised me. However, I saw the condoms as a small thin interface between life and death. Simple. I fully understood and began to timidly explain to our patients that there is no "safe sex" apart from abstinence. However, there is "safer sex." Information and changing of a few habits could save lives. I was much impressed with this simple concept.

I went to the local drug store and bought a few gross of condoms. The check-out clerk looked at me with interest. My own risks were in my mind. Was I unknowingly infected? Was I infecting Dan? I had better use some of these condoms myself. I did.

AIDS would become a disease to challenge healthcare systems throughout the world for years.

"Déjà Vu" is from this same experience. I recalled the near

meltdown at Three Mile Island, 10 miles away, in March 1979. I recalled polio in a friend of mine in grade school around 1952. While AIDS was new, and in fact our young patient's illness came before there was even a name for it, I had a sense of having been through this before.

AIDS was a holocaust of sorts in those days. There were too many funerals, but there came a time when the funerals slowed down and then stopped. Those who had been infected early on are now gone, but I still tend to dress in black.

1990

BAG LADY

I have a coat
long and full and warm
It closes in and keeps me round
It contains my world
        and there I savor
wonders and gifts
once lost to me
Tea, a cup hot and steamy
one in Styrofoam today
Tannic moisture that lingers
        on my tongue
Leaves steeped and weeping
        that turns to tea for me
Places warm and soft
like memory's womb
I settle in and watch
the prance and patter
from a cardboard crate
A biscuit with sugar and butter
        cozied in my pocket
for later, nestled there
next to Emily Dickinson's poems
to savor within the hidden folds
        of this grand and musty coat

WINDFALL APPLES

What genetics, XY
chromosomes
    blew them down?
Down to the ground
    with bruises
already turning
To be salvaged and used
only by early quick
    gathering
Only watchful eyes
like my grandmother's
Or an eagle's
would gather them
if left where the gusty
wind fell them
Where worms, bugs,
    and any variety of decay
would take the opportunity
To attack

DÉJÀ VU

It washes over me
The float, the flood
of grey, blue and charcoal
Picasso squares
Fish scales
I feel the pebbles, stones
Crustaceans of the narrow sea
at my back
Pointed, scraping
Fluctuating
Freckled trout and nymphs
on tide memory

Both "Sundance" and "Non-Webbed Feet Upright Housebuilders" reflect a time when Dan and I moved into a new house. And it was truly new, in that we were the first occupants. These poems were fun. The fossil-hunting archeologist in my psyche wondered about what we were building on top of and wondered who or what we might be disturbing. I have a preference for older houses, but do not have the skill or the knack of restoring and maintaining them. We have dear friends who have an old house from the 1700s, and I watch their "nesting" with great interest and admiration for all their skill and patience. George Washington is thought to have had breakfast in their house in October 1794 during the Whiskey Rebellion; they just need to document it. As I read my American history and look for Reagans, I have the small hope of stumbling upon it for them.

The real mystery is this: what do we really know about the history of the soil, the earth, and the structures of the dwellings within which we have chosen to live? On what archeological level are we living? And from what do we derive our happiness and success? Do we even know what happiness and success mean – at least for us?

The basis for "December Dream Wind" is a visit to my father on the first anniversary of my mother's death. My father is still cautious about death at this time, hoping that everyone is alright. To his credit he remained a fathering person despite the loss of his wife, and his own grief. It was in his nature to look to the welfare of others. One day when we sat talking, in a somber moment he looked at me and said, "I am so sorry that you lost your mother." He wanted me and my brother to be alright. He wanted our children to be alright, and he grandfathered them to the very end of his life. He was comfortable enough, beyond his own grief, to acknowledge ours in a way that I never expected. He taught us to the very end; he taught me when I didn't even know what he was teaching. What a silly daughter I was on so many occasions.

1991

SUNDANCE

Squared cubes of ice
Hit the glass of the second-story
window of a two-story colonial brick
with a view of the park
Shatter it
Heat and fire
    of the morning sun
Laser sharp
shards dance
on the dreams
of a sleepy brain
and carve out
the ache of hangover
    and collective memory
Lethargy of long lived
    years of sundance
from the gray dark
crevices
Rolling ridges like turned soil
rich and moist
Pain is removed
Scooped out as if it were
an old benign tumor
And the yellow star
the scalpel
Razor edged and keen
Bright with flame
Strong and healing
He steps out in a three-piece suit
Squints into the morning star
Squints
Steps onto the graves of kings
And attributes his Wall Street well-being
to a pulsating shower head

DECEMBER DREAM WIND

He knocks, taps on her door and she sleeping late, hears him ask:
Are you alright?

Some slight memory fear in his voice, some vocal cord readiness:
Are you alright?

His voice floats along on the same dream wind of her sleep-waking
    mind
with recollection of toy tractors
    cranberries and wrinkled
    Christmas paper, ironed
    and reused each year
    twine kept in a ball
    white snow floating sideways
blowing and tingling her face

A midwest farmer, wise and winter bent:
Are you alright?

Why wouldn't she be alright?
Of course, she is alright
Pink and daughterish
More awake than asleep
Now, she recalls:
She's dead, now a year

He's perking coffee
weak from small pinch-like scoops
He reuses it and boils it a second time
Yet it's weak
As if now his time of bounty is gone
Passed into memory
Buried
She awakes, fully now

and drinks his
pale brown coffee with him in
silence of morning

Later he will tell her how
he dreams more now but reminds her:
He always dreamed

NON-WEBBED FEET UPRIGHT HOUSEBUILDERS

There are no ghosts here
They must bring their own
or create them as they go
among concrete and carpets
But yet they hunt for ghosts
wanting to use the rituals
that would throw them out
They find instead a wild grape vine
that the bulldozer didn't
Honeysuckles now bloom
    where weeds struggled
      a month ago when they shopped
Two or four daisies sway
Love and love-me-not
Escapees of the landscaper
But there are no ghosts
and low
pressed tight against the earth floor
wild strawberries stir
with white round petal faces
with cherub-sized red berries
They peek waif-like
children refugees
Soon to be ghosts
that will not survive
the non-webbed feet
of the upright housebuilders

Some poems exist just for the beauty and imagination of creating the poem. "Watershed" is such a poem. As can be seen, I have created poetic distance by speaking of myself as "she" or "he", but my poems are not always about me and my personal experience. Some are pure imagination. Some are the result of stepping into another persona and imagining what it is like. The pleasure of creative writing and especially poetry is the freedom to create new worlds and live within them through various literary devices. "Watershed" was my own little word symphony.

Poetry is much more than expressing emotion. Confessional poets, such as Anne Sexton, moved us into a wonderful and worthwhile cathartic territory, but the novice poet should not be lulled into believing that these poets threw away all the conventions of poetry. There was still the concern for rhyme, meter, form, and metaphor and other devices literati.

"Watershed" was also one of those poems written in response to the itch that all artists understand. The hand starts to move towards the paint brush or the shutter. For the writer, words need to be written. For years I thought I wanted to be a painter, because this itch always seemed to start in my hands. I just didn't have that kind of talent, and soon learned that a pen and a journal were more satisfying scratches to my artistic itch.

I write my poems in longhand in a journal and then transcribe and revise onto my computer. There is a tactile nature to the process. One problem inherent in this approach is that I always seem to be about six journals behind in transcription. Although I have tried secretarial help, it just doesn't work, because the transcription point is also a point of revision. And oh, revision – perfection is thy aim! A poem truly is never done, and here probably lies the basis for poetic angst. I love editors, because they will say "stop" and really mean it!

1992

WATERSHED

The slow summer wind comes off
>   the mountain
Falls in long violin sound
Strings through all the trees
from the mountain's spine
Ridge rocks and jack pine and locust
Down the bass gullies of watershed
to the meadow lace
>   here below
Resonant long after it has
>   moved on
Pleasant warm recollection
>   in the frills of dress
>   ruffles of easy gossip
Of those pulling on gloves
and tossing concert stubs
>   in the crowded lobby

PRIMARY CARE

Two geriatric
recovering alcoholics
having their coffee
at first suspicion
But their old tan
seasoned hides
    cover long strong
    flexors and extensors
    abductors and supinators
    pronators
and cruciate
as they raised coffee to lips
gave lie to suspicion
Two retired farmers
at the stainless steel
diner on the main road
Retired by paved
roads and grown children
or government subsidy

If I walk out there
    and get hit by a truck
    that's one thing
You know what I mean
Now when I buy hamburger
I get the meat from "my" butcher
You know what I mean

And "my" mechanic
fixes my car, you know
What I mean

"My" doctor
I'll listen to "my" doctor

If I walk out there
   and get hit
   You know
Well, that's one thing

The almighty dollar
that's the other thing
The cars speed by
   too fast to be counted
A train passes
   beyond the paved road
Another train as they watch
And drink another cup of coffee

I liked writing "Primary Care", which was another poem of the imagination versus a description and interpretation of reality. Yet I must confess that, although imagined, it surfaced after having coffee and listening to the cadence of speech at other tables in a roadside diner. I liked these "tough customers." I must confess further that I have a habit of listening to the cadence of strangers' speech. Although I cannot hear the specific words, the tone and measure are always there. This casual speech is so uniquely human. I imagine this kind of language arising in stories told around a fire, whether by caveman or camper.

⊬═══⊣

"Who Owns the Libretto", written in 1993, is one of my own favorite poems. The poem questions ownership of information, and in an informational society this question has become crucial. I have never completely understood why the patient's chart is off limits to the patient. In a culture of rapid information exchange, this tradition of secrecy is curious. The poem arose in my imagination when I overheard a discussion about a patient's right to go to the "stacks" to find information in our medical library. The topic of the poem is now obsolete.

Oh yes, I understand that if you, as the nurse, have not documented "you have not done it", and I understand the need for communication between disciplines and shifts. I just have never understood the secrecy. I love using the proximal and distal language of medicine and nursing, but have never understood the secrecy.

Ironic! Now the Internet is *so* useful for accurate and inaccurate medical information. Irony now reigns.

If healthcare reform finally arrives in the USA, at the core of successful reform will be appropriate and confidential information exchange with the patient. I am not sure this will happen, as reform appears to be in the hands of politicians who know nothing substantial about the system, are reluctant to truly learn, do not even read their own favored bills, and are certainly disinclined to ask nurses like me and physicians like mine.

I am fortunate to be the patient of an enlightened family doctor who happily hands me a copy of my test results. He invites and answers my questions. You might say, "Well, you are a nurse, and this is one of those professional courtesy things." My response would be that no, I see him in action with other patients, and I suspect that this is the nature of family medicine.

At present the health insurance companies have a curious priority over the patient with regard to intimate information. The patient, in one way or another, "pays for" both the physician and the insurance. Isn't this rather like buying a book and having someone else keep it on their shelf and read it for you from time to time? It is curious. However, as my own family doctor demonstrates, the process can be better, and it doesn't take tons of bailout money and it doesn't take years of time. Catastrophic situations aside, it simply takes human beings acting reasonably. For educators and those who make curriculum decisions, healthcare could be much improved with more support for educating nurses and family physicians and less support for educating lawyers.

One inherent problem with the healthcare system and the political system in the USA is that too many of the legislators are attorneys. The very nature of their ingrained process is self-perpetuating, and puts them out of touch with the average citizen. Thomas Jefferson and George Washington, among other of our founders, were adamant about keeping the common touch in government. Ours was to be a government "of" and "by" the people, and that premise has long been lost in the USA.

1993

WHO OWNS THE LIBRETTO?

They browsed briskly though
the medical stacks
Text after text
Pushing page after page
He watched her quick movements
He held her grey coat
To allow her arm room
and give her space to breathe
She pulled from
shelf after shelf
Bent on her knees
Stretched up her arms
Then leaned back and sat down
Lifted her knees as in
stirrup for childbirth
Book after hardbound book
Looking for a gush of water
Found one
This one
Splash of a waterfall
Look at this one
Pointed him to it
The illness there
Their respirations now fast
The illness of their child
described with paragraphical details
Graphs and diagrams
Percentages and prognoses
They looked
Side to side
Held their breath
so as not to be caught
in their act
Not to be scolded

in their act of love
their moment of near death
The inner sanctum
stacks on stacks
of well worded knowledge
of medical texts
An act of suspicion
that would confirm   or deny
what the doctors told

LONG HOSPITAL STAY

From the end of the corridor
A four year old looks at the tunnel
of movement, trays and carts
Gondola meetings
through guarded eyes
Through a venetian blind
    Squeaky water clean
    white soft-soled shoes
    Drawers and doors
    and needle caps
    Rings, beepers, and bleeps
He pulls them open and closed
Adjusts them to keep out
the flow of alcohol and betadine
Or to let it all in, sliver by sliver
He just watches
Watches for snags of limb and branch
Shadows of wolf and bear
Tiny sentinel who moves
an invisible cord of golden twine
that calls upon flute and chime
We would forget what he had
seen and heard
We would forget
that he was a child
And he falls asleep finally
on a rickety river raft
with hand still pulling
to protect his dreams

There is a part of me that still lives among the tall grass and the wild-flowers on the slope of the Missouri meadows where my brother and I found all the arrowheads. For me it is a healing place. The sight of fossilized fish tails in stone on the edge of Galway Bay is also healing, at least for me. I feel good when imagining these places and these things. I suspect that everyone has special places and special things, but as nurses and physicians we don't know these small details about our patients. And in what context would we learn of such intimate specifics? "Medicine from the Wood" is about these intimate and healing specifics and a desire to come to the bedside with a medicine from the earth itself.

1994

MEDICINE FROM THE WOOD

Wooed by juniper berries
and promises of bitter persimmon buds
we remain long in this wood
I carry all the proofs
to your bedside
like a radiologist
whose specialty is artifact
In a tightly woven basket
grey slate with fossil fern
Soft mounds of moss
    still warm
Fish tails in stone from Galway Bay
Pine cones
Pine resin
Hickory nuts
Hikers' orange peel
And silvery spider web
And the kiss of a mayfly

FEATHER AND CLAW

Birds fly in and out
and take my soul
on their wing
Midnight nurses
with penlight bones
Hollowed flutes
I hear the rattle
of their coming
and their going
I feel their beaks
sharp tongues
feeding on me
They take piece
by small piece
in the hours
before the sun
I am amused
with wonder at this leave
taking of me
Escher fins and fishes
of air and sea
I beg aphasic
to leave something

The action in "Orphans" never happened. It is a composite of various things that did happen, but is a poem of the imagination. Watching my father with animals around the farm often gave me pause. I recall him often with the horses. My brother was always there to interpret for me, although his own activity on the farm and in the forest was often just as dangerous. The fording of creek beds at the time of flood or in the time of drought was a tricky business, but necessary in order to get from one place to another. There were no bridges across every stream. Indeed it was important for my father to know the land and the creek "like the back of his hand." To get back across the creek, he also needed to watch the sky and the clouds to anticipate the weather that would or would not allow his return home with two children.

Years later, when I was an adult, my mother confided in me that she always hoped that I would stay at home with her rather than head out with my father and my brother. Two things concerned her – first, that I would never learn the work of the house, and secondly, that I could be hurt. However, she kept her silence and never said anything. She seemed to understand a child's need for drama and excitement, especially there in the backwoods.

I hope that "Orphans" relates some of the fear that came from the idea of being an orphan. Life was so fragile, as demonstrated both by my grandfather's story and by what I observed every day.

Cortney Davis and I met in 1993. Our writing, thoughts and work were taking place in the same Zeitgeist, and a partnership for two books was born. In 1995, I wrote "Snow on an Old Landscape." That year, Cortney and I were thrilled to have the University of Iowa Press publish our book, *Between the Heartbeats: poetry and prose by nurses*. It was an international first. (*Intensive Care* would follow in 2003, again published by the University of Iowa Press.) Cortney and I had admired *Visions of War, Dreams of Peace* by Lynda Van Devanter and Joan A. Furey (published in 1991 by Warner Books, New York). I was so proud – of myself and my fellow nurses – in 1995. And now we are raising our voices, from our life experience as well as from the 24/7/365 bedside experience. My joy was – and continues to be – as crispy clean and unique as a snowflake.

1995

ORPHANS

I wouldn't be so sure of it
Not again
The horses through the high water
across the creek in panting struggle
Lathered and thirsty from the effort
Drinking from the stuff
that caused the sweat
I held my breath
an inverted prayer for success
My father held the reins
and my brother watched
with greater skill it seemed
than me, his eyes placing each delicate hoof
before it disappeared into frothy water
Tense movement of his head copying our father's effort
I would never trust the water again
or the forest or the trees
The earth that until now had belonged to me
Had been stardust when I kicked my bare foot
Had been champagne when I upheld my mouth
in the mists of April rain
It opened an abyss now to bury my father
to take him, the wagon, and the wild-eyed
horses down to a creekbed that had no end
Their eyes were innocent and terrified
Holding the two emotions in one round
window of heaving pulling animal flesh
My brother was older, old enough to know
His peripheral glance was a shout
Silent and swift in the morning air
His ten-year-old hand motioned me back
One leg break in the lead horse
and we would be orphans
I would never be so sure again

I would learn to watch, feel caution
and fear, loneliness that can come in one
bone-shattering moment

SNOW ON AN OLD LANDSCAPE

Dedicated to nurses like Cortney Davis, Ted Deppe, Jeanne LeVasseur, Veneta Masson, Joyce Renwick, Belle Waring, and others who are writing up a storm and changing the landscape of language and nursing practice.

We hold out our hands
and feel the snowflakes fall
One after the other, different
and new, to cover an old landscape
We never thought it would look like this
We scatter to the front of the room
to read poetry, nurses with words
suddenly, but we proceed with caution
on soft-soled mercy feet
Ears, eyes, and hands watchful
We know how Alexander Graham Bell felt
We know the first snowflake on an infant's cheek
And we know the difference between rain and tears
And we bask in this snowfall
open our mouths to it
and laugh as if it were all sun

The relationship between doctor and nurse, and especially between medical student and experienced nurse, is rich with ambivalence. For the medical student the experienced nurse can be a walking encyclopedia of knowledge, and within the complicated hierarchy of medical school, the nurse can be a reputation saver and a skill maker for the medical student. A first-time experience with an intravenous needle on the night shift can be traumatic.

I love the keen sheen of idealism in the medical student. The nurse, usually female, can be sister, mother, grandmother, or lover, and in fact the relationship with male medical student sometimes becomes that of wife, as with some of my friends.

1996

ON BEING PASSED BY A CLASS OF MEDICAL STUDENTS WHILE SEATED

Does one call them a flock?
A gaggle, a class, a school?
I feel their draft
on my calves, my feet
Air stirred at gastroc
Frantic pace
I feel them first
by this cold stir on my legs
as they pass
Pass from class to stairwell
Down, down to lunch somewhere
Chatter of
    number of points
Fragments of conversation
    see ya later
runs into
    it was a challenge
and
    I thought last year
Words fade into the stairwell
Fall down the stairs
like a nun's practiced rosary prayers
dropped in a hollow cathedral
    Do not speak to us of the greatness of poetry
    Of the torches wisping in the underground
    Of the structure of vaults upon a point of light
    There are no shadows in our sun
The cold stir ceases
when the last one closes the door
We will meet tomorrow in the clinic
and on the floor
    Slowly the ivy on the stones
    Becomes the stones

This nurse stirs reluctant bones
moved by some stiff crucial ligament
Her first task will be
to water the flowers on the ward

1997

SEMANTICS

I bathe my thoughts
Turn them, roll them in a bed bath
and apply clean white sheets
on the one side
while the body holds on the other
I pull the freshness of cloth
under the body
Pull the fabric smooth and tight
and fold and wrap the corners
I bathe and collect my thoughts
in this tidy movement
around a comatose body
I keep out all meaning
This unidentified body
admits no visitors

1

9

9

8

HE DOESN'T DRIVE ANYMORE

He stands there on that spot at the corner
He looks autistic but he's not
Every day he watches the spot
He watches a discrete space
the size of a ripe watermelon
the length of a grown man's foot
He watches a moment in time
He tries to go back – pull back
from that oblong globe of time
A concrete space on the road
where his foot hit the brake – too late
A fractured second – three hundred yards – too late

THE PARKING LOT DISEASE

Their steps are slow and cautious
Side-steps as if walking on ice
The man and the woman cross
from the door of the restaurant
to the door of the maroon car
Their shoulders are curved
in tense consideration
of a slippery substance
I'm squinting but I can't see
        But
                Stop-this-is-August
Just a grey bone-dry tarmac
Scent of oily residue long gone
The temperature is eighty-eight degrees
The time is mid-afternoon
Broken hips and medicare
Senior citizen discounts downtown
Fragility of inflation and late December

"Labour Day" is an attempt to recall in poetic format an event from my childhood. I will say more about this event later, in my discussion of "Preschool", published in 2003.

1999

SUN AND MOSS

I
The late evening spring sun
falls on my daily skin
like a warm, clean blanket
Crisp, full, abundant
fresh from the clothesline
        Fluff it out
        over the baby on the gurney
        with promises
        White-shoe-scared-rushing
        with promises
        Time, the angry knot
        of a dark sun
        No promises
        at the back of the neck
        withdrawal of light
        No promises
The close of evening sun
heals every spot it touches
A bright and willful start
unaware of spots untouchable

II
The moss held to stones
like mother to child and child to mother
The sun flickered past
each day at noon
like shutters and windows
Soft held to hard
and hard to soft
Sun held to window
like reflection on water

The moss held to stones
like flesh to bone
and bone to flesh
Water of sea, earth and air

HOME VISIT PROGRESS NOTE

I consented to join the celebration
holding onto policy and procedure
He said:
> *Nettie and I would often*
> *Have a glass of wine on Sundays*

Nettie, I learned was a sub-category nickname
Her real name was Nettles
He would laugh out loud and say:
> *Nettles!*
> *Yes you would have liked Nettles!*

Her real name I didn't know
but I guessed at Netta.
Could spend all the late summer afternoon
in entertainment by learning the nicknames
of all the citizens of his small coal town.
Could chuckle-spend it but wouldn't
in deference to policy and procedure
He said:
> *We would use these glasses*
> *on a Sunday – here use these!*

Not goblets, but bold blossoms resting on a tall stem.
The tobacco-rich red wine filled the elegant bowl,
then our taste buds, ending with a warm wash down our
throats.

As the liquid faded down to the last vague petal
in a smooth titration, the ease of our laughter rose.
Sage, fennel, marjoram, and oregano gone to seed
outside.
Hollyhock, sunflowers slipping into repose for fall.
The attic odor of sage pushed through the screen door,
> over the smooth-grain floor covered by worn
carpet,

into the yellow-bright small kitchen where we
sat.
I resisted a look at my watch with the swift moving
second hand,
with which I weekly counted the beats of his failing
heart.
I resisted a reflection on policy and procedure
Written by attorneys with high salaries and low expectations.
He said:

This is good for you, isn't it?
Improves the appetite
Good for the heart, they say

LABOUR DAY

It was on labour day
The lake was silky with silence
Still and calm as flat fabric
No swimmers awade
No boaters astride
No oars flashing – stirring
No – no – nothing
Men on horses
Boots, saddles, roar
Dust – sweat – shrubs, tall grass
Tree branches parting
to let them through – *he's loose!*
He killed her – shot her
    Dead
                His own daughter
He's running somewhere
Shadows fall across the cloth
spread for our picnic table
            He's running somewhere
         We'll find him – through the field
They found him
         Shot himself – in the head
Voices of farmers yelling
from neighbor to neighbor
passing the news
The rain started to fall
calling off the hunt
The rain became heavier
The aftermath of fear
a ripple of a raging stream
Disbelief a deep cavern
of seething black water
The lake serene – still
quiet witness.

2
0
0
0

SEEING MY GRANDSON FOR THE FIRST TIME

Now – I have seen you
I am reminded
of someone I know
Miracles are small
One
at-a-time
Two
Three
Four
Five
Six
Seven eight
Nine
Ten fingers
Ten pink toes
Soft eyelashes
Paper fingernails
Window pane eye-lids
Moist smell of baby dew
First vision of an angel

A golfer's voice came from a back room at Tralee Golf Club: "White House evacuated. Pentagon on fire." On that sunny warm afternoon in Tralee, Ireland, I had been reading and writing a few lines while Dan played golf. "World Trade Center!" I slowly rose from my books and my tea and headed towards the voice. Two or three golfers were huddled around the televised photos on Sky News in the back of the Club. The smoke was rising from one of the towers of the World Trade Center. The first report was that a small plane had accidentally hit the World Trade Center. One news reporter asked about the controllers: "Are they having problems?"

But what of the Pentagon? "Stock exchange is closed."

More golfers, mostly Americans, came in off the course and crowded about the television. Dan and his foursome were probably coming up on the sixth or seventh green at some distance from the Clubhouse. It was not realistic for me to walk out. I would watch and wait.

"Another plane has hit the other tower!" New York was on fire! Smoke was billowing on the television screen. I stared. I was paralyzed with fear. In April we had just celebrated our second grandson's first birthday. Our daughter, her husband, and our two grandsons live just outside New York City! My sister-in-law and her husband live in Connecticut and work in the city. They were just going to work in New York. It was morning there.

I wrote things down in my journal. World Trade Center. White House evacuated. Pentagon on fire. Another plane hit the other tower of the World Trade Center. Airports closed within, into, and out of the United States. Our country is being attacked.

Other golfers were coming in. Phones were jammed and busy. A nice young waiter at the Tralee Club helped me to make a call to our daughter, but the phone was busy, continually busy, time after time.

I went out to the ninth green which circles back up to the Clubhouse and saw Dan coming in. He said that I was standing there sobbing. I don't recall when I began to cry, but realized at that point that I was – and had been.

We were soon to learn that the fire at the Pentagon was from a third plane. It would take a few minutes before we could grasp the fact that a fourth plane came down in Pennsylvania, near Pittsburgh, near home. We listened to the reports of cell phone calls getting through, to and from the passengers. Once they learned from the phone calls that their plane was being used as a missile, they purposefully sacrificed themselves and brought the plane down. There was speculation that the intended target was the White House or the Capital Building in Washington, DC. No one really knew.

With the help of Dan's caddy and his wife (a nurse, by the way), we called our daughter again and again, and finally contacted her around 2.30 in the morning, Irish time, from the caddy's home phone. We changed our plans and secured a room in a local bed and breakfast and headed back to Galway the next morning. We knew the lay-of-the-land and we knew people in Galway.

There was nothing to do but walk from pub to pub, from television to television, and watch the news and call the airlines and see when we could get a flight home. We took turns calling Aer Lingus. It would, of course, be days. From pub to pub the story on Sky News was the same. Dan and I do not usually hold hands as we walk about, but on those days in Galway we did.

We, of course, finally left Ireland and got back home. Each and every passenger on our flight either overtly or covertly made a mutual pact: "We will not let this plane be used as a weapon." When we landed in Baltimore, applause and cheers sounded throughout the plane. On our drive north towards Pennsylvania, towards home, we saw numerous signs along the highway, most of which said "God Bless America."

Our bucolic suburban existence had been shattered. We would never be the same again. We still feel, today, much less awkward about expressing our love for each other and for our family and friends. I say this now to all my dear friends. I love you and I am grateful for the richness you have given my life. To our daughter and our grandsons and our son-in-law, I love you and I loved you before you were born, I love you now and I will love you into infinity.

2
0
0
1

A WELCOME TO A SECOND GRANDSON

Your big brother and I walked
downtown for ice cream
Chocolate chip mint
Polite, seated at a table
while your mommy labored

Along the way we found
feathers, stones
and prickly "porky-cones"
One dime
and a friendly gray tiger
kitten
napping on a sun-filled
New York village day

Your dad relieved and your
mommy needing rest
A cell phone call to Opa
We welcomed you
Your big brother offered animal cookies

FOLDING FRESH LAUNDRY

When my mother died
we went through her intimate belongings
and threw them out in black plastic bags
My father, her best friend, and me
I was astonished at the chaos
in the last toss with life and pain
Drawers were stuffed with lingerie
Odd shelves and cupboards
stuffed with unfolded linens
Sheets, pillow cases, laundered,
unfolded and unordered by color, stripe or flower
No apparent category could we see
except for the pattern of pain
and the texture of fatigue
Fluffy flowers sprung from crevices
Patient paisley grew from hidden nooks

2002

VITAL SIGNS OVER TIME

Paper evidence of a life
    Over time
A life recorded in bills paid
and commitments met
Taxes, bar bills, postage
Progress notes
TPR and BP
A litany we sang in nursing school
temperature, pulse and respiration
Blood pressure and signs of life
Thank you notes and until-
we-meet-agains
Logged and dated
Credit card and cell phone
Beeper, pager, call bell
Nurses recorded
for all the world to see
Hiding there in plain sight
Thousands of nurses
Bills paid, payroll deposited
Bed made and floor dusted
Trach suctioned, oriented times three
    Over time nurses
Alert and responsive, on overtime

SECURITY

Sprawled belly down
on his parent's bed
Too old for naps
he seeks retreat
from the summer sun
    To think
        To think
            To think
The fluffy comforter cool
to sweaty face and arms
arms wide, fingers curl
    Floating
        Floating
            Floating
Legs thin with muscle
suspended on a cloud
Fluffy as cumulus
As distant as cirrus
Six-year-old aloft in dreams

I am often asked about my favorite books and who are my favorite contemporary writers. I, too, like to ask this question of my fellow writers. The question is impossible to answer because, like most writers, I read everything from the cereal box to history, science, mystery, and, of course, poetry. I especially love the poetry of Cortney Davis and Ted Deppe and others such as Jeanne Bryner and Veneta Masson and all my other fellow nurses. Cortney takes words and bats them out of the ballpark and the words slam past you with the mach one force. I am a fan of everything she writes. Ted reaches back into history and the human psyche and pulls words forward into a new world and creates a new climate and a new history. And I am a fan of every word he puts to paper. The novels of Irish writers – John Banville, Dermot Healy, and Edna O'Brien – are an inspiration. By this I mean that the writing is so rich and powerful that, as I read through their novels, I keep my journal handy and find myself stopping to write poetry, and then going back to the novel again. So the answer is a long one, one which I could not even start to answer here.

Des Kenny of Kenny's Book Shop and Gallery in Galway, Ireland, sends us books, as part of his book packet scheme, on a regular basis. Although less regular in these days, as Dan and I head towards the financial restrictions of retirement, I rejoice to get some of the Irish writers as soon as their books are out.

While I am at it, I will include two other frequent questions. How much do you read? And when do you write? A day without four hours of reading and/or writing is a slump day, and I become a cranky addict without my fix. As to the second question, I write all the time and I carry a journal with me everywhere – in my pocket, my purse – but absolutely all the time. Like a photographer with a camera, I am afraid that I will miss something.

Alright, there is one more question that surfaces. What advice would you give to new writers?

The answer is so obvious that it is usually overlooked:

1 Read good literature.
2 Write.
3 Revise and revise and revise.
4 Read more good literature.

5 Write again.
6 Revise and revise and revise.

A photographer friend says it another way: Crop and crop and crop again. Writing groups can be really good, if you are lucky enough to find a group with which to work, but be sure that they keep the focus on the writing and the quality of writing. Too often groups can disintegrate into formless and unfocused oblivion.

I love new writers and new poetry. One of my greatest pleasures is seeing the poetry come into *PULSE*, an e journal edited by a physician, Paul Gross, and the *International Journal of Healthcare Humanities*, edited by a nurse, Cheryl Dellasega, out of Penn State University's College of Medicine's Department of Humanities. I am a poetry editor for both, and I thrill to the new voices and the new work.

⊹≕≕⊹

Although the poem "Security" seems to be about a boy, it really recalls the first time I read a novel, *Robinson Crusoe*. I changed the protagonist's gender in order to give myself some literary distance within the poem. The *Crusoe* was an abridged version for children that belonged to my brother. I sneaked into the house and hid in his room, sprawled on his double bed, and read it from beginning to end. The room was summer cool and he had the oldest child's advantage of a double bed. This was pure sprawling luxury.

Reading, still, is a naughty exercise of stealth for me. There is a logic to this. Reading and "book learning" out of necessity had to take a back seat to the work required on a farm. I grew up with that. Planting, growing, and harvesting were at the mercy of the soil and the weather. Reading and writing were not. Reading and writing were functions of unessential luxury, the forbidden apple. I still have a sense of consuming an exotic forbidden fruit when I read. I love it!

Subsequently, *Robinson Crusoe* has over time remained one of my favorite books. Other books that were childhood and young adult favorites include *Chee and His Pony* (by Florence Hayes), *The*

Adventures of Huckleberry Finn (by Mark Twain), *I Capture the Castle* (by Dodie Smith), and *Magnificent Obsession* (by Lloyd C. Douglas). I am also a reader of Eavan Boland, Robert Frost, Seamus Heaney, Paul Muldoon, and Wallace Stevens.

As a child, I had a sense of ownership of Mark Twain. He grew up in Hannibal, Missouri, just up the river – the Mississippi River.

I once argued the point with a colleague that as a child I was greatly influenced by the Mississippi River, as I was born 20 miles from it. She couldn't buy this – that the influence could be so strong when the river was 20 miles away and I really had no experience of living on or splashing in it. It is a curious argument, but the influence is true. Recall that I am on a farm about 20 miles away, but our stories and books are of Mark Twain and his Tom Sawyer and Huck Finn – and the River. We were those sweaty fence-painting children. We were overly busy, as only children can be, with making our own adventures and solving our own mysteries. We relished Mark Twain and his muddy river.

I wish I could go back to the low spot in the meadow – rich with arrowheads and conglomerate rock. We conjured up bows and arrows and painted horses. We ran with the wind through Queen Anne's Lace and wild white clover and found hiding places near the stream in the woods. We solved mysteries by overturned stones and tracked footprints on recently travelled paths. We looked for caves and hidden treasure. Samuel Clemens was our very own.

I even broke down a bridge across the mighty Mississippi. My mother was diagnosed with adult-onset diabetes. And later, as a nurse, I came to know that she had diabetes early on, or at least she had gestational diabetes around her pregnancies. My brother and I were both big babies, which is a sign of diabetes or potential diabetes in the mother. I weighed in at around 10 pounds or more. The night before I was born there was a great storm and the bridge over the Mississippi at Chester, Illinois, blew down. My birth story was that I was so heavy that I brought the bridge down getting here. It is a funny story but I wonder – and regret – how much my mother suffered giving birth to big babies in a back bedroom with nothing but my father's hand for anesthesia.

By the way, I hated that story. From day one I was considered overweight. I have been dieting ever since!

2
0
0
3

PRESCHOOL

The neighbor wipes her mouth
With the hem of her apron
Shouts across the pebbled garden path
From her kitchen door to my mother's porch

Rain clean and steady on the gray stone
Rain sweet and slow on the kitchen window
Drips and ripples on the pane, imagining
                    Shot . . . killed his daughter . . .

I push closer into the softness of my mother
Smell flour, apples, and the heated pulse of fear
Her arm comes around and finds me
                    Then . . . killed himself . . .

She nudges – nudges me back, pushes me
Into the house, she stretches to hear
The rain taps. The day suddenly raw.
                    Cold. Her hair now wet

Silence – when my brother comes in from school
Whispers – when my father comes in from work
Candles. Flowers. Perfume.
                    Prayer worn, wooden pew

Listening. Imagining. Awkward. Listening.
                She was pregnant . . . can you imagine . . .
Wax form of a young woman's body in a long box
Rain clean and steady on the gray stone

As a nurse I cannot help but read these poems at this distance and reflect on what seared my childhood's heart and soul – and seared me so painfully that perhaps I was drawn to the helping profession of nursing. "Labour Day" from 1999, a few pages back, and "Preschool" from 2003, are both about the same defining episode. Curiously, "Labour Day" suggests what my father was doing and "Preschool" records where I was with my mother. Although they are works of the imagination, the poems are about an all too real episode of incest, subsequent pregnancy, and the resultant homicide and suicide.

As an adult, I know now, of course, what "that" was all about. The remembrance of my thoughts as a child, as recorded in the poems, is of alarm, fear, and chaos. At the time of the episode, I was a preschooler or thereabouts, and I didn't even know the meaning of words such as sex, incest, homicide, and suicide. The adults were acting funny. The funeral of the adolescent was solemn and sweet, but the grief of those in the church was shaped in what I knew as shame and guilt. It was that feeling that I had when I had accidently broken a Sunday dinner plate, but worse – much worse. The silence in our small community was knifelike, and the pain and fear of living within the mystery, at least for me, was extreme.

In the back of the church, the dead adolescent's older sister sat in a well worn pew, and spoke words I could not hear. I strained forward to hear from a crouching position I had taken up under the pew some distance from her. Never mind the dust and the crushing of my go-to-church dress. Her face was red and tear-stained and her shoulders shook. I heard words of father and sister and problems between father and others. I couldn't hear the words. I smelled stale furniture polish on the pew and waxy candles and sweetheart roses from near the coffin. Confusion was mixed with smells of death and sounds of sobbing. In those days and in that cultural place, parents took their children to funerals, and indeed took them everywhere they went. I would not know the word "babysitter" until years later. Although I was knowledgeable about animals' deaths, I had not known human death until this funeral.

I don't recall hearing about or going to a funeral for the father.

All I knew was of mommies and daddies and babies after they

got married. This experience was not fitting my small view of the world.

I watched my father for a sign of information. I watched my mother for a sign of information. There was nothing. My brother went about his life as usual. My cousins went about their lives as usual. Our neighbors and my uncles and aunts went back to work and about their lives as usual. I followed their curious lead.

No one ever explained to me what had happened. I put it together piece by piece, year by year. Not so curious then, in retrospect, that I would eventually become a pediatric nurse? As a pediatric nurse, I knew from my very gut and tried to put into practice with children, even babies, the idea that a young child will cooperate with medical procedures when told simply and calmly two things – first, what is happening, and secondly, that they are in a safe place. I have now read and have had neurologists explain that the comprehension of language is developed long before the expressive use of language.

KVO*

Up early
The neighbor's porch lights
   still blaze
    Beacons to a warm morning off
  in July

  Call light
    to my lazy heart
      that this morning, at least
I am first on my cul-de-sac
to watch the drip of the slow rain

The sweet water drips into the rusty
  hole of a septic gutter
    Falls onto lilac leaf
      Drains down the point
        to the dusky-end
         Falls onto parchment
       stubbles of a 2 × 2 patch
      Brown brittle torch
    of begging thirst
  of planet earth
I reposition myself in old scaly wicker
and monitor the rain all morning long

---

* KVO means Keep Vein Open; it is a common practice to maintain a slow drip of intravenous fluid to keep the vein open for future or emergency administration of medication.

2004

NURSES' FEET

One day post bunionectomy
Reading Darwin, recuperating
   keeping dressing dry
   popping pain pills
Wondering about sedentary wings,
the strength of Wedgwood and bone
Reading – writing – refraining
from the onset of pain
Elevating, contemplating
   my evolving bunion,
Rudimentary digit
formed from genetics
and a nursing career
Driving 50 diseases backward,
ward nursing on mercury wings
   and an enthusiastic thirst
   for jogging, running, dancing
high heels and gastroc gender tension
Pain surgically relieved – soon

THE RETURN OF MEMORY ON THE SHORTEST DAY OF THE YEAR

Whose woods these are
I think I know
Cedar sprouts and shrubs
Rock ridge and deep
double ditches
Back road stone chips

Past the persimmon tree
   Past the silver poplar
      Past the barn pond
         Past the catfish pond
            Through the wheatfield
               Through the corn stubble
            Under the oak tree
         Over the acorns
      Under the salt lick
   Over the winter dust
Round the garden gate

Running all the way
Up the field-stone-steps
one-at-a-time like a puppy
returning home
Onto the wooden porch
panting at-the-door
I think I know

2
0
0
5

LOSS

I saw a woman come to stand
on the beach in the cool of morning
She looked across the strand, pointing
and gesturing as if a small child
stood at the hem of her gray skirt
Talking and pointing for the child to see
some object in the distance, across
the water and through the mist
I, myself, at a distance
but curious – I watched her
As she turned to go
I saw there was no child

I would not be one of those nurses who married a medical student or resident. Lust never developed into life-engaging visions of a shared future. Dan, my life partner, would be an award-winning pharmaceutical representative with a sparkling smile and sparkling eyes and a cheerful temperament – he was a born salesman. We could talk the same medical language. He was Irish Catholic and I had always been drawn to Irish Catholic men – fun and filled with stories. I loved them!

One of his mentors, Bob McAndrew, would introduce us to Ireland, and from that point onward our life would be lived between Ireland and America. They both received awards such as "President's Club" numerous times, and other titles such as "Distinguished Sales Rep." Bob died much too early, and "The Burial of a Distinguished Sales Rep" was dedicated to him. His eccentric spirit was a silent and generous one.

The poem was fun to write, with the attempts to weave in words from Robert Louis Stevenson's "Requiem" and at the same time include words from the song "Danny Boy." The poem took a long time to write, and I happen to like it a lot.

Although I submitted the poem to *Wild Onions* with enthusiasm, I was surprised that it was published, because it seemed too personal. I am thrilled to include it in this collection.

THE BURIAL OF A DISTINGUISHED SALES REP

Dedicated to the memory of Robert McAndrew:
On the day he was buried, we learned that he was just a man after
all – but an uncommon man of uncommon love and generosity. He loved to
sell. He loved and protected his daughter.
He loved Ireland. He loved people. Travelling, talking, and selling
were his hobbies as well as his career. He is sadly missed – on both sides of
the Atlantic.

On the green hillside, near the summit   *The pipes, the pipes*
behind the chosen plot, in the purple shadow
the grave digger cleans his nails with a penknife
A cigarette dangles impatiently from his mouth
while mourners listen to the sweet clear
sound of a blind daughter's acappella
of sun on mountain heather; she recites

the pipes are calling

Home is the sailor, home from the sea
The November night rain has created
clingy mud that suctions to our shoes

from glen to glen   ·

We make tracks into a train station
We drink his beer and hear his stories
at his daughter's dimpled invitation

and down the mountain side

Tales of a salesman's treks
Tales of Ireland. We laugh, we cry
And the hunter home from the hill
Floors of marble, murals repainted
in green, gold, vermilion
Remade into a restaurant
Travelling now transformed   *the summer's gone*

2006

ONE BRIEF SUMMER IN CHILD'S TIME

All of us, doctors and nurses
Social workers, all of us degreed,
Nine years old and he learned us
Like the spring wind learns the willow
Each stem and turn of leaf

Sleep apnea and multiple co-morbidities,
MR; to our credit we learned
To believe in his capabilities, within hours
Of this trach, finger over his airway
    The wind attendant on the solstices
    Blows on the shutters of the metropoles
He learned he could talk; he learned
To pick up the phone and page me; charm,
Engage me. I would become his gatekeeper
And move his check-ups along, more time to play

He learned the other patients, sharing the ward
Learned when they were likely to die, learned
Life was made of minutes, seconds, tumbling
Like fall leaves in a storm. Still wonder about IQ,
Winter, the result of caring – and the results of tests

Emergency surgery late on a Friday night is a worst-case scenario, as any nurse can tell you. Dan, who was already being worked up for abdominal pain by a gastrointestinal surgeon, had his colon perforate on a Friday night. A friend happened to stop by our house at the time, grabbed the keys and drove us to the hospital. Dan was going into shock in the car. My question as we went into the ER was "Who is on call?" His surgeon, the surgeon who knew his story, was on call. I knew he would be alright – a friend just happened to be there at an unusual time, and the right person was on call. Ducks were in their row.

It was a long cold night deep in the month of February 2006. He went into the operating room within less than two hours after perforation. But once out of the operating room, there was trouble getting him off the ventilator. There was sepsis. Pain. Cardiac complications. He was two long weeks in the intensive-care room. He survived!

There would be subsequent surgeries, ileostomy reversal, wound vacuums and hernia repairs. He would return to work, to Ireland, and to the golf course. While in surgery, I developed the habit of talking to him – hence this poem and the allusions to Shakespeare's *Midsummer Night's Dream*. Literature was at work and was at least healing for me while I waited.

2007

LONG FRIDAY NIGHT EMERGENT SURGERY

You are bold walking through these dark woods
late on Friday, nearing midnight
I fear deep, soft undergrowth
No path but some deer tracks
to take you along the stream
if we shadows have offended
to lead you near the well
While the moon is on the thin,
Pray, your swaying lantern stays aglow

Pray, you're close enough to hear
the expressway's loud sea sound
Recall, we so often complained about
the loud sea pulse on a summer's night
through our window – *think this and all is mended*
you have slumbered here
Pray, listen, for direction
through – or pray, you are so far in,
the loud sea sound will give direction out

"Summer's Over" is a poem that I could not have written in 1984. Every bit of it is so real and scalpel true down to my very bone. The poem is not made from imagination but from what was left at the end of the summer of 2007. Seven relatives came from Ireland. Dan and I were thrilled with their visit as he was not ready to travel to Ireland yet. It was the first time in 75 years that someone in Dan's Irish family had travelled in this direction to America. Years ago, on our first trip to Ireland, he made an initial connection, and he and his cousin have become the keepers of this family torch. We have the hope that the connection will hold through future generations, and with the Internet and easy communication we know that the connective torch can be carried on faithfully.

Our young grandsons had visited at the same time, and after they had gone I saw a fresh footprint, from the chlorine of the pool water and spilled juice boxes, on the kitchen floor. There were also stubborn fingerprints from milk and cookies around the door and on the refrigerator. I chose not to clean.

In 2007 my father had died at the age of 95 years in Missouri. He lived as long as Charles Carroll and longer than Ronald Reagan. His uncle, James Reagan, died at the age of 105. My dad would have said of all of them, "Tough customers." And now I say that of him – "one tough customer."

We buried him on an 107-degree day beside my mother in a high meadow cemetery next to Reagan's Chapel Methodist Church in Missouri. An era had passed, and my brother was now our patriarch. We would move forward to new destinations, some known and some unknown. I would be transformed, but nothing like I could have imagined in 1984.

No, I could not have written "Summer's Over" in 1984.

2
0
0
8

SUMMER'S OVER

The bright sun has brought a red, green,
and golden harvest to our smudged door
with finger prints of cousins and grandsons
Reluctant to swipe it clean, look around
We find footprints on the floor, a summer to remember
And not wanting to be entirely clean and clear
of this brief season, we wax and wane
Search under the scratchy leaves for a red tomato
Finding none, watch the squirrel prep his store
    We savor old wine
    Consider the pleasures of a new neighbor
    Loss of a father and burial on the plains
    in one hundred and seven degrees
The bright sun shines on
Still time to prune the trees
Caulk around the door
Prepare for bitter cold

I still have not figured it out, you know, this business of war and peace. Guess I never will. From reading the Bible, I sometimes think that God and his inspired scriptwriters have never really figured it out either. Yet I do know that every human being needs – and probably has – something that they would die for.

And for me, it would not be poetry but it would be the right to write poetry. For that right to speak and the freedom to write, I would surely die. Above all else I would lay down my life for our daughter and for our grandsons, for Dan, and in general for my family. In "Peacemongering", I toyed with the idea in the context of Robert Frost who surfaces often in my poems. Is having the gun an act of peace or an act of war? There is no conclusion, of course. Even the most peaceful among us have a striking point where the match will become the flame – or in some cases where they are the match and others become the flame. Consider Ghandi and Martin Luther King Jr. No one person knows their own or another's striking point, but I believe that the point of flame is always there, somewhere within us.

2009

PEACEMONGERING

Is it true that Frost wrote poems at night
in the kitchen with a revolver on the table next to him?
Uncomfortable with the truth that might come tumbling
unexpectedly from his words? Did be become impatient
with all the peacemongering? Do we all want, at some time,
to rise up fighting and turn words into bullets and give up
on prayer and plowshares, study and sacrifice?
                              And like Frost
do we look and sound so predictable
and undangerous? Faithful farmers
watching fields of brown wheat and yellow corn,
pacing intensive-care cubicles in isolation gown;
Walking through the green clearing,
caging free-range chickens, corralling colts,
holding back, fearful of great risk. Fearful of fields in flame

DESTINY/DESTINATION

A strange thing for us to do
but we were in a foreign country
with stiff new passports in our pockets
And strangeness was more than welcome
The elderly hitchhiker looked tame enough, slightly boggy
Moist with smells of new mown sweet hay
        and mothy wool
Once in our hired car, his brand of English, if it was that,
was not ours. He sucked in great heaves of air and sighed
        out grey round stones
Sounds that rolled forward over our shoulders,
        as his eyes stayed on the road
He watched the windshield from the shadows in the back
seat. We pretended some kind and nodding comprehension
        but we never understood
And yet he signaled effectively enough
for us to stop, open the door and let him boggle out
at the crossroads, some five miles later
Brown woolen hat tip and toothy smile
Some gratitude was expressed
some agreement on a fine day

Afterword

Some of my later poems are about loss, destiny, and different levels of discomfort as well as common daily problems such as foot pain and memory loss. Any seasoned nurse might chuckle at the aptness of these concerns and might throw in some descriptive back pain to make sure there is a full understanding of what nurses do. Nursing is hard physical and mental work. Staff nurses working the wards do not have the luxury of retreating to a desk where they can sort out their decisions. These nurses thinking on their tired feet are the heroes of the healthcare system.

There is the corresponding privilege of being with other human beings at their most vulnerable and intimate moments. With this privilege, nursing becomes a sacred trust.

I thank you, each and every patient for the privilege of being your nurse.

I thank you, each and every reader. I hope that the profession of nursing is a little revealed here in all the caring – and confusion – that is there each and every day. I have seen minute by minute and day by day the compassion of nurses, doctors, and other healthcare providers. I have been privileged to spend my career in this environment.

I, like most nurses, started out in school where I was taught the white starch of professionalism and the rules of not getting too involved with one's patients. Although I respect the basic wisdom of the instructions, I have learned that human nature functions otherwise. We are all in this world together. Curiously, the function of professional distance confronts the nurse with the concept that we share the same earth, sea and air space. Although we have different backgrounds and experiences, we are at the bone all human. Perhaps I learned this lesson early with my family around the coal oil lamp, before the magical electrical lines came strutting through the woods. I certainly know I learned the love of stories there in those dusky nights together with my family. To be a nurse is to know daily, intimately, and repetitively – 24/7/365 – we are in this together, all over the world.

Title Index